A mind of one's own

Digby Tantam
Clinical Professor of Psychotherapy and Honorary Consultant Psychologist,
The Centre for Psychotherapeutic Studies, The University of Sheffield

Sue Prestwood
Counsellor for people with autism and Asperger syndrome,
Community Health Sheffield

The National Autistic Society

The National Autistic Society

Published by The National Autistic Society
393 City Road
London EC1V 1NG

First edition published 1988
Second edition first published 1991
Second edition reprinted 1998
Third edition first published 1999
Third edition reprinted 2002

ISBN 1 899280 09 X

Designed by Cottier and Sidaway Design Partnership

Printed in Great Britain by Crowes Complete Print of Norwich

Preface to the third edition

This small booklet has proved to be a useful introduction to Asperger syndrome for parents and people with Asperger syndrome. As more and more people are recognised as suffering from this socially disabling problem, it affects a much broader group than was previously thought. We have therefore increased the scope of the book to cover issues about marriage, getting older, and siblings. We have also taken account of recent research on Asperger syndrome and our own experience in counselling people with the all too common emotional disorders which may be caused by having the problem.

Contents

Introduction

This booklet is about that group of more able people with autism sometimes described as having Asperger syndrome. Although the term Asperger syndrome will be the main one used throughout, most of what is said will apply equally to those more able or high functioning individuals who have, perhaps because of their childhood history (see section on diagnosis), received a diagnosis of autism.

The more able person with autism or Asperger syndrome will be referred to as 'he' throughout. This is because men and boys considerably outnumber women and girls in the condition, by a ratio of between 6 and 10:1, although it seems possible that women with autism are less likely to be diagnosed. This may be because women tend to have much better social skills than men, and women with Asperger syndrome may therefore be more able to conceal the extent to which they experience social or emotional problems.

The person with Asperger syndrome is a person with a disability

Cause and associated problems

Autism and Asperger syndrome are most usefully considered as a disability, such as blindness or deafness, rather than an illness, such as 'flu'. This disability can arise from a number of conditions which affect the brain, as well as from malformations of the brain which are present at birth.

Since an underlying illness may cause other problems, it is to be expected that autism will often occur in association with other disabling conditions. Autism is much more common in people with a learning disability (that is people with an overall psychological impairment and not just an impairment of social functioning); and it is associated with clumsiness and with epilepsy.

What is autism?

The autistic disability is not easy to describe in words although most people who have dealings with people with autism get a strong sense of something being 'missing'. Lorna Wing has suggested that the disability can be detected most easily in what she calls the triad of social impairment (Table 1).

Table 1	Wing's triad of social and language impairments
1	Absence or impairment of two-way social interaction
2	Absence or impairment of comprehension and use of language and non-verbal communication
3	Absence or impairment of true flexible imaginative activity, with the substitution of a narrow range of repetitive, stereotyped pursuits.

Language abnormalities alone do not make a child autistic although they may contribute to the social disabilities that a person with autism inevitably has. However, the abnormalities of social interaction, interest and play do seem to be shown by all people with autism and Asperger syndrome, and together may constitute the essential disability.

The social use of language

The more able person with autism or Asperger syndrome will not, by definition, be learning disabled. Neither is he likely to have serious language problems persisting after early childhood since these are associated with lower ability. However, muddled speech and the use of neologisms (made-up words) may sometimes occur and more seriously, so may problems with the social use of language.

People who are not autistic modify their vocabulary, their tone of voice and the amount they speak to accommodate the listener. Adjustments are made without thinking for the listener's age, social status, sex and emotional state (evidence that people with autism or Asperger syndrome are less well able to judge these characteristics will be considered later).

People with Asperger syndrome do this much less well, and indeed, if they do it at all, it may only be because they have been taught the 'rules'. Accordingly the person with Asperger syndrome may be too terse, or conversely, may talk for much too long about topics of special interest to him. He may interrupt or cross-question an older or higher status person. This may be a source of embarrassment or ridicule. It may lead to the person with Asperger syndrome being shunned by others, or to the more sensitive person with Asperger syndrome becoming apprehensive about situations where unstructured social intercourse is likely to occur. This may lead to social situations being avoided or to conspicuous anxiety about them.

Unfortunately social situations almost always demand an adequate understanding of these subtle clues and no explicit set of rules could possibly be drawn up to cover every contingency. One person with autism, who was very mildly disabled, did well in an interview at a public school until the end when he asked how old the headmaster was. The same boy maddened his parents by coming into a room where they were, and positioning his chair outside the family circle. At times they thought he did this deliberately and, perhaps after a while he did defiantly place his chair as near to the door as possible, but in truth he had no real conception of where to put a chair so as to appear to be part of a social group.

Non-verbal communication

Interpersonal problems could arise either because the person with Asperger syndrome is failing to interpret unstated indicators of age and status, or because he is not able to modify his behaviour to accommodate them. Actually, both seem to occur. People with Asperger syndrome seem less able to interpret non-verbal cues than people who are not autistic (scientific evidence about this is presented later), and also use them less.

A good example is the difficulty that people with Asperger syndrome have in using context, especially non-verbal behaviour, to modify a verbal statement. Jokes and ironical statements are consequently taken literally, sometimes with embarrassing results. Exaggeration, metaphor and confidential remarks all present similar difficulties to people with Asperger syndrome, and, if misunderstanding is not to result, are best avoided unless kept at the simplest level. By contrast, obvious jokes, humorous exaggeration and puns may be much appreciated.

People with Asperger syndrome also have difficulty in making their speech colloquial or in leaving things implied but unsaid. Consequently they often appear ponderous or pedantic. Occasionally people with autism are good mimics (more usually less able people with autism) but in these cases the person with autism usually reproduces exactly what someone else said in the same tone of voice. People with autism have considerable difficulty in impersonating others, that is in inventing what someone might have said.

It is often difficult to tell what a person with Asperger syndrome is feeling from his facial expression or tone of voice, and the latter may have a flat or querulous quality. Other abnormalities of non-verbal communication are considered in a later section.

Self-presentation and social judgement

People with Asperger syndrome can be taught some social and conversational skills, but these are not the only adjustments that are required in social situations. It is also essential to have a reasonably accurate understanding of how another person feels and thinks in order to judge how to present ourselves: to deceive, to charm, to flatter, to seduce, to sympathise and so on. We also use knowledge about self-presentation to be able to judge other people's motives, to know, for example, when to trust them. People with autism do not have these abilities and suffer from a serious excess of honesty and trust which exposes them to exploitation.

People present a picture of themselves through their conversation as well as through their personal appearance and that of their living space. The living space of a person with Asperger syndrome is often either impersonal or a jumble of objects which have accumulated either randomly or as part of a collection. There is no attempt to make any impression on other people. Clothes are similarly nondescript. In fact it is very rare for a person with Asperger syndrome to buy them, even if they are quite capable of buying other things, such as records. People with Asperger syndrome generally have no concept of fashion or style.

Many children with autism have abnormalities of movement, including odd postures, repetitive movements, odd but habitual ways of doing certain common actions, and stiffness and lack of fluidity in movement. These may be especially apparent in the person with Asperger syndrome. He may have considerable difficulties in acquiring motor skills, particularly those which, like riding a bicycle, require posture control. Odd or stereotyped movements may contribute to the poor presentation of the person with Asperger syndrome. Odd postures can cause people to keep their distance, but people with Asperger syndrome may be able to learn to monitor and suppress them. People with Asperger syndrome can also be taught to postpone the rocking, muttering, whistling, chin-tapping or other 'stereotypes' which give them comfort. Unless the person with Asperger syndrome is given some permissible situation in which these movements can be indulged, however, they may start to carry them out in the street rather than at home. These oddities produce embarrassment for parents and may alienate some people, although they rarely give serious offence.

By contrast, asocial behaviours, such as yawning, grimacing or inappropriate smiling during conversations, may be less indulgently received. Therefore, if a person with Asperger syndrome commonly uses them, it is a priority to help him become aware of them and of their effect on others. In attempting this it is important to remember that the normal meaning which would be attributed to the behaviour is lost on the person with Asperger syndrome. Hence statements like, 'You should pay more attention to your father' or, 'You must show respect to your teacher' are not going to change the behaviour of the person with Asperger syndrome because they are not going to be understood.

Play, interests and hobbies

Children with autism show an impoverishment of play which may be complete in the most disabled person with autism. The play of more able children with autism or Asperger syndrome typically involves ordering, grouping and contemplating objects. Play is usually solitary although children with Asperger syndrome may be passively involved in play by other, more dominant children.

Ordering may also intrigue children who are not autistic. They sometimes like to make collections just as more able children with autism or Asperger syndrome. The solitary play of the child who is not autistic differs from that of the child who is autistic, because it includes enactment. Children who are not autistic will imagine that they are train drivers, or mothers, or doctors, and will put on special clothes and a special voice to show that they are not being themselves. While children with autism hardly ever seem to do this, it is not entirely accurate to say that they lack imagination. One girl with autism, for example, made up names for all the household machines, and said they were the home of different races of tiny people to whom she would attribute responsibility for her naughty behaviour. She also used to like her father to describe an imaginary journey they took together down beneath the lawn in the back garden. Some children with autism or Asperger syndrome may also write stories or poems.

As the child grows older, play metamorphoses into hobbies and interests. Most children's interests are influenced by their friends and are allotted only so much time as can be spared from social activities. They are often carried on as part of a group or as a member of a club. People with Asperger syndrome frequently have interests too, but they are private, often idiosyncratic, and absorb a considerable amount of attention.

These special interests may involve routines as, for example, the boy who loved to arrange a toy car- track in a certain position and then watch it; they may also involve collections of things or of memorised facts, or abstract study. Collections are often very narrowly restricted, eg maps, books about a specific topic or photographs. Facts to be memorised are often very circumscribed. One 65 year old man memorised the addresses of juvenile courts and was 'bored to tears' with the addresses of other courts. Other facts memorised by people with autism we have met are the top twenty, jockeys and winning horses (quite common), the names of carrot species, rose varieties, Beatles memorabilia, the lives of the Mitfords, bus routes, the livery of Great Western trains, Dewey decimal classification numbers, capital cities and their tallest buildings, astronomical facts, boxing records, the dimensions of cathedrals, maps of towns and dates. The subjects of abstract study have included non-verbal communication, psychopharmacology, toxicology, astrophysics, biology, the history of World War II, archaeology, the Bible, and chess puzzles.

Most of these interests involve systematisation, something that seems especially important to people with autism of all ages and all degrees of disability. Many of them also involve people but in a reduced or remote way. Either a very few people were involved (the Beatles, the Mitfords), or some physical measurement of people was involved. Many people with Asperger syndrome like to read the *Guinness Book of Records* possibly for this reason, and one person with autism, when asked to describe his uncle, said that he had a 50 inch chest and a 40 inch waist.

Sometimes the interest allows a glimpse into the struggle of the person with Asperger syndrome to make sense of people and their behaviour. Two people have been very interested in the Arthurian legend, because they wanted to be a 'parfit, gentle knight' like the knights of the Round Table. Another person read thrillers because he could not understand how the criminal could lie and then be found out. This man could understand the facts of the story but could not follow its plot because the motives of the characters were opaque to him. Many other people with autism or Asperger syndrome have similar difficulties with fiction and may only be interested in factual books and documentary films for that reason.

Callousness and lack of empathy

People with Asperger syndrome have difficulty in understanding the feelings and thoughts of other people and consequently they lack empathy. This makes it easy for the person to become selfish and, unless external checks are placed on this tendency to impose his routines on the family, the person with Asperger syndrome may become a tyrant. One adolescent with autism ruled his parents' life to such an extent they were afraid to go out, had to shop surreptitiously, spent a considerable amount of time cleaning because their son was thrown into a tantrum by dirt, and at every meal had the nightmare of persuading him to eat more varied food. People who are autistic, like people who are not autistic, modify their behaviour according to its predicted result. Most people with Asperger syndrome learn early on that hurting others is followed by the most serious consequences and usually act on this rule. However, a few people with Asperger syndrome are violent towards others. This violence may have a frightening quality as a person with Asperger syndrome is not restrained by a show of fear or the look of appeal on his threatened victim's features.

Rage may be prompted by exposure to a special aversion, as in the case of a man who attacked women and girls who sang at a certain pitch. Rage may also be prompted by frustration over the change of a routine; or by emotional reactions to situations, such as bullying and teasing. In such an example a person with Asperger syndrome lacks the necessary social understanding and verbal or social skills to deal with the situation appropriately.

Sexual and property offences are rarely committed by people who have Asperger syndrome. When they do occur, it is often because of the lack of social understanding of the person concerned. The most common offence is one involving some degree of violence which may, very rarely, lead to death. The aggression may be indirect, through fire-setting or the sending of dangerous items through the post, or it may involve a direct attack. This level of violence is not reached immediately; there will have been some rehearsals of the act, and a great deal of cognitive rehearsal. Rumination about particular episodes when the autistic person was the subject of violence, or a preoccupation with a feeling of powerlessness or loneliness may precede the violence by many months.

The victim of violence may not be the person who has caused offence, but someone who is vulnerable and unlikely to be able to defend themselves. Sometimes, the victim will be in the same category as the person against whom the aggressor has a grudge. Sometimes, the victim will be a stranger who provokes an unwelcome emotion in the aggressor.

Routines

The more disabled a person with autism is, the more they are bound by routine and the less able they are to adapt to change. Routines about eating, about what is eaten and how it is prepared, about going to bed, about getting dressed and going out as well as routinised interests do sometimes cause difficulty in the households of more able people with autism or Asperger syndrome.

Routines seem to have the function of reducing anxiety and uncertainty. They may become less obtrusive if other steps are taken to calm fears. One girl with autism who loved to sing became more and more importunate about her singing lessons with her mother. She insisted they took place at the same time every day, even interrupting her mother's conversations and physically dragging her to the piano. For her part, the mother always tried to cut the lessons short and would skip them if she could.When the mother began to write down a lesson time and duration every morning on a board in the kitchen, her daughter's behaviour became much more reasonable. It was even possible to plan to miss the lesson on occasional days.

Interest in people

Kanner originally described children who were aloof from others and, children with autism were assumed always to be cut off from other people. Indeed, many psychoanalysts took this as the starting point for an understanding of autism. However, observations of children with autism have shown that they make the same number of approaches to each other as do normal children in a group. These are characteristically brief approaches, much less likely to progress to an interaction, and are quickly followed by withdrawal. But the fact that many children with autism initiate these approaches indicates a normal level of interest in other people. It does not follow, however, that children with autism are interested in the same things about people as children who are not autistic.

What does seem to distinguish people who are autistic from people who are not autistic is that interaction is apparently much more likely to be unpleasant for the person with autism. Consequently the offer of interaction is much more likely to repel a child with autism or Asperger syndrome than a child who is not autistic. Those of us who are not autistic rarely consider the possibility of failure in social interaction, unless there are exceptional circumstances, such as ringing someone on a bad, long-distance line or talking to someone in a foreign language. However, failure of social interaction is a regular occurrence for the person with autism or Asperger syndrome and this is one possible explanation of why social interaction may be repellent.

This explanation would fit in with some of the known facts about the relationships of people with autism or Asperger syndrome. One well established observation is that aloofness is more common in younger, and in more severely impaired and disabled children with autism. These groups have had less opportunity to learn social skills and are therefore going to have the greatest difficulty in managing social interaction. Aloofness could therefore be a way of avoiding situations which provoke anxiety.

One of the many controversies surrounding the treatment of children with autism has concerned how far to intrude upon their aloofness or passivity. A social approach to an aloof child with autism will provoke behaviour which seems to be due to anxiety; rocking, gaze avoidance and so on. However, persistent intrusion can, under some circumstances, increase the likelihood of future social interaction by the child with autism, and decrease the amount of asocial behaviour, such as rocking. The behavioural hypothesis, which proposes that the person with autism or Asperger syndrome is in conflict between wishing to interact and experiencing an anxiety due to a failure of interaction, could explain these findings.

Social intrusion increases the anxiety of the child with autism at first, leading to more asocial behaviour, but if the intrusion leads to some interaction which can be successfully maintained, the child's anxiety drops. When the interaction ceases, the child has gained in social competence and lost some anticipatory anxiety for the next episode of social interaction.

The more able child with Asperger syndrome, assisted by parents and teachers, can generally achieve sufficient social competence in early childhood to be able to stop avoiding social interaction. However, the same factors which affect the self confidence and outgoing nature of a child who is not autistic also seem to influence the child with Asperger syndrome. Some children with Asperger syndrome continue to be shy and rarely initiate social interaction but others may become 'active and odd' to use Wing's terms. Many more able children and adults with Asperger syndrome fall into this latter category. Since they do not discriminate much between strangers and friends, these people may be ironically too ready to get into conversation with strangers or visitors on occasion.

Marriage

Some more able people with Asperger syndrome do get married. Indeed it may only be as a result of difficulties that arise here that the disability comes to light. These may appear almost from the outset as the adjustments needed to share their life fully with someone may prove a lot more difficult than envisaged. It may be a long term realisation by the partner that the person is not going to change as they hoped as the relationship progresses. Alternatively it may be that the initial adjustments go well enough, but when other pressures arise and more demands are made, the person with Asperger syndrome finds that they can no longer cope and withdraw in one way or another. Such pressures could include the birth of a baby or children becoming older and their needs becoming more complex. Unfortunately the levelling of blame and accusations of selfishness from their partner only add to their anxiety and thus tend to increase their rigidity and exacerbate the problems.

Counselling from a relationship counsellor who understands not only the difficulties but also the strengths of people with Asperger syndrome can be helpful. For those who are able to appreciate their partner's good points, such as honesty, faithfulness, lack of hidden agendas, and tolerate their more difficult ones, such as obsession with routine or an inability to give empathic or emotional support, marriages can work well enough. For others however, the lack particularly of the latter quality can become too great an obstacle and the marriage breaks down. The partner can be left feeling angry and let down that they never knew that their partner had this difficulty or was genuinely unable to change. People in such situations are now working to set up support initiatives. More information can be obtained from The National Autistic Society.

The person with Asperger syndrome may also be left feeling angry, frustrated and/or depressed at their failure in the relationship. Alternatively they may feel bemused or angry towards their partner for their 'unreasonable' demands or complaints, being unable to recognise their own inadequacies from their partner's point of view. Counselling from a counsellor who understands Asperger syndrome may help them to begin to address this, learn from it and begin to move on.

People with autism or Asperger syndrome are vulnerable to emotional problems

Early adolescence brings particular problems; much more initiative and responsibility is expected and the new dimension of sexuality is added. Many people with autism reach puberty late and, even then, may not experience sexual attraction. However, the majority of people with Asperger syndrome do have sexual feelings in adolescence and many of these use masturbation as a means of releasing sexual tension. Few people with autism have recovered sufficiently from their disability to be able to engage in the degree of social reciprocity necessary for a long term intimate relationship. Many people with Asperger syndrome have never even dated anyone. Sexual frustration is therefore common during adolescence. This may lead men and women with Asperger syndrome to respond to inappropriate sexual invitations from other people. They also feel a great deal of pressure to 'be like everyone else', or what they perceive as 'like everyone else'. For example they often interpret TV 'soaps' as a true reflection of normal life and usually believe all they are told by peers who feel the need to brag about their own sexual prowess and conquests. This may compound their difficulties, making them even more vulnerable.

More disabled people with autism do not achieve enough social competence to be at risk sexually and, in this respect, are less affected than the person with Asperger syndrome. This may lead to more able people with autism or Asperger syndrome paradoxically having more emotional disturbance than the less able. Emotional disturbance is especially likely to occur in the teens and early twenties. Conduct disorder (emotionally driven misbehaviour), depression and anxiety may begin in adolescence and are probably more common than in non-autistic children. One survey did however show they were no commoner than in adolescents who were not autistic but who had social difficulties.

Leaving school may also be a time of stress since, there is a further increment in the expectations that other people place on the adolescent. Removal of the structured environment of school may show up previously unremarked social difficulties. A common pattern in the person with Asperger syndrome who has been academically successful is that the first job is consistent with examination results but only lasts a few months. It is followed quite quickly by another job of a less responsible nature. This lasts less time still, and there follows a succession of less and less responsible jobs, often resulting in unemployment. If the parents or their professional advisors do not appreciate the social disabilities of the person with Asperger syndrome, this apparent deterioration may be wrongly attributed to a severe mental illness, such as schizophrenia or even dementia. It is likely that the emotional problems of people with Asperger syndrome occur for the same reasons as the emotional problems of people who are not autistic; strain on a person made vulnerable for lack of a secure attachment to other people. Attachment is difficult for a person with Asperger syndrome to achieve but it is probably made easier or harder by different kinds of upbringing. It is undoubtedly important for the person with Asperger syndrome to feel secure in his parent's affection.

Other people's reactions

The emotional security of a person with Asperger syndrome is only one example of the way in which other people's reactions can have psychological repercussions for someone with Asperger syndrome. Another example is the effect of victimisation (teasing and bullying) on people with Asperger syndrome. This may have long-lasting consequences because the person with Asperger syndrome thinks over and over again about the unfairness and the cruelty of how he has been treated. Teasing is often stated by people with Asperger syndrome as the reason for their emotional problems, or as a justification for aggression.

A note for professionals on the physical and mental health of the person with Asperger syndrome

There is a greater likelihood of having another physical problem if you have Asperger syndrome, and these associated conditions often need treatment in their own right.

People with Asperger syndrome who are not born with an associated condition are more likely to develop epilepsy than others, but this may remit again in adolescence. There are no physical conditions which develop in later life more commonly in people with Asperger syndrome than in the general population.

Evidence of neurological damage is common in autism but it is less common for a definite neurological syndrome to be present. The EEG may be abnormal and up to 25% of more able people with autism or Asperger syndrome may had had fits although few will have regular fits or require anticonvulsants. Psychological testing may demonstrate a marked superiority of verbal over performance scores, by contrast with most less able people with autism who show the opposite tendency. However, the difference may be absent or in the opposite direction.

Mental health problems do occur more commonly in people with autism. Some may be related to the brain condition which is thought to cause autism. Severe mental illness ('psychosis') may be one such problem. People with autism or Asperger syndrome appear to have a higher risk of psychosis than people who are not autistic. This excess used to be attributed to schizophrenia in one study but it is now thought to be mainly due to bipolar affective disorder (manic-depressive illness). Both mania and depression take the same form in people with autism or Asperger syndrome as they do in people who are not autistic but the content of the illness may be different. One manic man with autism was preoccupied by a new bus route which would link up all the places in North London that he liked to visit. A man with autism who was very depressed threw himself into the Thames because he despaired of persuading the Government to abolish British Summer Time; another refused to speak because he believed that he might give away secrets to the IRA.

Other mental health problems might arise because of the stress of having autism or Asperger syndrome. These include depression, anxiety, obsessive-compulsive disorder (recurrent, resisted thoughts or behavioural rituals), and drinking problems. Conduct problems may also occur in childhood or in adolescence. The same treatment that work in people without autism, often work in these situations, too. One recent development has been for counselling to be used to help people with some of these problems. Counselling cannot cure the underlying social impairment, but early experience suggests that it can produce considerable social and emotional benefit and that this may reduce the apparent severity of the core problem.

It is worth considering an emotional problem whenever there is an otherwise unexplained deterioration in the behaviour or social function of a person with Asperger syndrome. People with Asperger syndrome may not always express distress directly. They are unusually sensitive to change, and they may therefore experience loss particularly acutely. Others may be surprised at how much the loss of another person may mean to someone with Asperger syndrome who may not have previously given any clue to the extent of the attachment that they felt to the person that they have lost. Depression is less likely to lead to a suicide attempt than in a person who is not autistic, but it may. Conduct disorder may be serious enough to require secure hospital treatment.

Having realistic expectations of a person with Asperger syndrome helps

Level of expectation

Having expectations of a person with Asperger syndrome which are too low results in an increase in disability. As a consequence the person with Asperger syndrome may fail to learn or to put into practice skills that are within his grasp and, if social expectations are correspondingly low, he may also develop more asocial routines and stereotypes. People with Asperger syndrome are capable of change in their social abilities, indeed many of the more able do become less disabled, progress being made well into adulthood. This development can be assisted by gradually increasing the expectations of the person with Asperger syndrome.

Too high an expectation does not have a facilitatory effect, but leads to failure or to recrimination. It is too much to expect of most people with Asperger syndrome that they will become completely independent. Table 2 gives an indication of what can be expected in more able adults, at least in those who have needed psychiatric help. People with Asperger syndrome are usually capable of learning to look after themselves in as much as they can shop, cook, clean and travel but they may need supervision of their self care as well as occasional intervention to rescue them from a difficult social situation.

Table 2 Social adjustment of 46 adults with autism

No contact with a friend in last year	70%
No sexual relationship for more than a month	78%
Unemployed	85%
Never married	98%
Resident in hospital or with parents	76%

As already stated these statistics relate to people whose difficulties have been severe enough to need psychiatric help. There are others who perhaps because they are not so severely affected or have had more appropriate support at key times, have muddled through, perhaps being regarded as eccentric or odd but nevertheless managing a higher degree of independence. Because in the past such people have been less likely to be referred or come forward for diagnosis there are no figures that we know of, to indicate the numbers who may fall into this category.

Because of wider ranging diagnosis and also such factors as change in work patterns more of these people are coming to light. Unlike years ago there is now very little chance of starting a job when you leave school and remaining in it until you retire. Even if you do not have to leave one job, eg because of redundancy and look for another, job descriptions change frequently and flexibility is the keyword. For the person with Asperger syndrome who needs routine, predictability and for things to stay the same, this is understandably very difficult. The more demands that are made, the more anxiety increases and the more inflexible or unable to change the person becomes. It may be at the point, where the job they have been doing in a certain way and often quite successfully for a number of years ceases or changes, that their difficulties come to the fore and perhaps for the first time may become overwhelming. Much support and understanding may be needed to help the person understand and come to terms with what is happening. They may need support in developing realistic expectations of themselves and where possible in reducing or breaking the changes down into manageable proportions, and establish new coping strategies.

Education

Many children with autism require special educational assistance. However, educational authorities have differing policies about this. A special school for children with autism may be provided by the local authority. There may be a special unit in a school for children with disabilities, or children with autism may be placed with children who have other disabilities. These placements may all be unsuitable for the child with Asperger syndrome whose intellect is developing at least as rapidly as his peers.

Some able children with Asperger syndrome may not receive any special educational provision because autism is not suspected. Estimates of the proportion of people with Asperger syndrome who never have schooling outside the mainstream very from 50% to 80% in the UK. A recent study by Ehlers and Gillberg (1993) of children with Asperger syndrome in mainstream schools found a ratio of at least 36 to every 10,000 and a further 35 per 10,000 whose difficulties could be classed within the wider autistic spectrum. Children with Asperger syndrome in normal schools are very frequently bullied but may be surprisingly successful in examinations. A few are able to go on to higher education. Whether or not a particular child would benefit from special schooling or not depends a great deal on local circumstances, particularly on the amount of help available from a local school. There has to be an understanding both of the child's social difficulties and of the sometimes patchy nature of the child's skills. Although one very bright 11 year old child with autism gained entrance to a local grammar school, he eventually went to a comprehensive school. There the headmaster was willing to provide a more flexible curriculum for him, accommodating more of his special interests in computing and tolerating more of his idiosyncratic learning habits.

Independence in adulthood

While many people with Asperger syndrome need sheltered accommodation and occupation, they have a greater need for independence and achievement than the less able person with autism. This often means that current provision for adults with Asperger syndrome is unsuitable. The right balance between supervision and independence may be difficult to achieve.

Awareness is slowly growing that many more able people with autism or Asperger syndrome than at present may be able to succeed in open employment. For this to be possible they need to be given the appropriate on-site training and support, and have well informed, supportive managers and work colleagues who, once they can understand the primary disabilities, can value the person's other attributes.

People with Asperger syndrome have qualities and skills like everyone else

It is important not to forget that, although the social handicap of autism affects almost every aspect of life in society, there are many other skills and aptitudes that a person needs. These, the person with Asperger syndrome may have in abundance.

Because of their interest in sameness, people with Asperger syndrome are often punctual and orderly. They are often conscientious and are not satisfied until the job is properly completed. If their work overlaps with their special interests, people with Asperger syndrome bring to it a considerable accumulation of factual knowledge although not necessarily comprehension. In a few cases, a particular aptitude underpins the special interest. This often results in the person with Asperger syndrome having outstanding abilities which are prized by other people. People with Asperger syndrome with a highly developed memory for pitch have become successful piano tuners, for example.

What is it like for parents?

Effect of behaviour

The parents of people with autism remain responsible for their children for much longer than a normal child and often have to face behaviour problems which are especially stressful, such as constant wakefulness at night, wandering, screaming attacks, food fads and aggressiveness. It is interesting to note that in a study of the causes of stress in families with severely learning disabled children the two most significant were identified as 'behaviour problems' and 'night time disturbance'. These rated higher than features like 'multiplicity of impairments' and 'health problems' (Quine & Pahl, 1985).

In the early years at least, their child may seem indifferent to them. In later years it can be very difficult to achieve the right balance between 'letting go' thus giving the child the independence he needs and retaining the appropriate level of involvement that he needs for his well-being.

Delay in diagnosis

Often it is the mother who first notices that there is something wrong with the child. She may initially either receive well-meaning reassurance from her husband and general practitioner which may only serve to make her feel more alone, or conversely, be told that she is making a fuss about nothing. Further delay in diagnosis is common, especially in the child with Asperger syndrome whose disability is less obtrusive. A fear of either inflaming guilt or hopelessness or kindling inappropriate optimism may be one reason why doctors still delay. Usually, however, parents have already concluded that there is something seriously wrong with their child and would welcome an open discussion of the diagnosis, aetiology and prognosis.

Furthermore, fighting for their child's needs to be recognised can be exhausting for a parent who is already experiencing difficulties in caring for their child. Finding out too late, some of the ways in which they could have been helping him or he could have been helped had an earlier diagnosis been made, only adds to their own feelings of failure, guilt or inadequacy.

Parents' feelings

The realisation that all is not well with their child or receiving a diagnosis can for many parents be a kind of bereavement in which they need to grieve for the 'normal child' they have lost along with the accompanying expectations. These may include level of achievement, possibly grandchildren and so on. This may involve the normal grief reactions of despair, denial, anger, blame, guilt and so on. However because their child is still very much with them, parents can experience guilt about these feelings and may need reassurance that the feelings are perfectly natural. They may possibly also need help in working through them in order to fully accept the child they have, with all his strengths and abilities as well as his problems.

Sometimes, because of their child's other abilities, parents of a very able person with autism or Asperger syndrome may explain their child's difficulties away perhaps regarding him as being very shy. Parents may then find it difficult to accept that there is a deeper problem when others, such as teachers or even the person with Asperger syndrome themselves, suggest this is the case. If acceptance comes it can bring with it guilt that the problem was not realised sooner or a feeling that perhaps the problem had been suppressed subconsciously because they had not wanted to see it. However the person with Asperger syndrome may in fact, in a desperate desire to be 'normal', actively seek to cover their difficulties and not confide them to anyone.

Most parents of children with any kind of disability experience guilt about their child's condition. Early clinical descriptions suggested that children with autism had abnormally cold parents, but as more clinical experience has been gained, this has been shown to be clearly untrue. Even so, many parents believe that, since their child's disorder is essentially one of a difficulty with human relationships, it must be due to themselves not giving enough of the correct emotional responses to their child. The considerable strains of bringing up a child with autism, especially when there is often very little reward in the way of responsiveness from their child may provoke parents to behave less tolerantly or less effectively than they would like, so exacerbating guilty feelings. Emotional upset in parents, marital stress, and angry recriminations with doctors and other professionals, may all occur.

Meeting other parents

Very often there are no simple practical solutions but the opportunity to talk about difficulties and their own reactions may relieve feelings and enable new strategies to be considered. Meeting other parents can be particularly helpful and there now exist many local society groups, affiliated to The National Autistic Society (NAS) and Branches of the NAS, which organise meetings and provide assistance to families. Membership is also open to professionals, and to people with autism or Asperger syndrome themselves. Readers interested in knowing more about the work of the NAS, the address of the secretary of their nearest local group (who can give information about activities), or obtaining information about conferences and study days should write to: The National Autistic Society, 393 City Road, London, EC1V 1NG or ring 020 7833 2299.

Coping with autism is made easier if the social isolation that parents often feel can be abolished. Meeting other parents either at conferences or local meetings can help in this respect.

Attitudes of other people

A child with autism makes unusual and prolonged demands on parents. This may cause parents to feel isolated from other parents and other people in general. A number of factors can combine to bring this about. Simply being too tired from caring and trying to balance the rest of the families needs and just not seeming to have enough hours in the day can be two. Also, parents almost all worry about their children, and many experience guilt although neither may have any justification in fact. Consequently they feel uncomfortable about attempting to socialise or take their children out in public. Other people who see the child with autism or Asperger syndrome behaving strangely, but who cannot see that the child has a disability, may contribute to the parents' distress and guilt by openly making censorious comments.

Parents who have more than one child with autism or Asperger syndrome may be particularly affected. Sometimes marriages can break down under these strains.

Respite

Respite care, where available can be helpful in such situations. This can have benefits for the parents allowing them space for themselves and each other and allowing them to come back to the task of caring with their batteries recharged a little and perhaps with a clearer perspective. It can be beneficial to other children in the family who can perhaps receive some uninterrupted attention from their parents or simply have a break themselves from their part in the caring.

Families and perhaps particularly mothers can experience guilt over even considering this option. But it is true to say that usually it is not only them but the child with Asperger syndrome who benefits in the long run, even if they may find it difficult at first. This can be in a number of ways; less stressed parents, wider experience, a wider circle of people who can care for him and understand his needs and so on.

Education

Decisions about education may be difficult. Parents, if they decide to keep their child in a normal school, may regret this decision when their child is bullied. One mother recounted how her child had regularly come home from school with his jacket torn and covered with other children's spittle. On the other hand the more able child may have less opportunity for achieving both academically and in terms of meaningful social contact if educated with less able peers. He may blame his parents for the special education that he feels has both disadvantaged him and given him an additional stigma with which to contend.

Aggression

Bullying may not be all one way. The child with Asperger syndrome may take out his feelings on younger school children, or on younger siblings, often because he lacks the ability to explain or deal with his feelings in another way. Aggressiveness may be a particular problem in adolescence, and the mother is often the target. It is often unexpected and can be fierce. One 14 year old, whose mother did not have the dinner ready, pulled her breast so hard that the skin tore. This level of aggressiveness is rare, and is probably indicative of an emotional disturbance complicating the autism, but when it does occur it is particularly difficult. Medical treatment of the child or adolescent may be required or, if this is ineffective, separation from the family.

Understanding autism and Asperger syndrome

Some of the current early intervention programmes for children with autism, such as the NAS EarlyBird Project are laying an increasing emphasis on helping parents to understand autism and how their child views and experiences the world around him.

This approach seems equally valid for parents of older children or adults, having several potential benefits. These include lowering feelings of guilt, shame and rejection by their child, as they gain a better understanding of why the child behaves or reacts as he does. Also because they gain understanding about why he finds a situation difficult or reacts in a certain way, they are more able to intervene or react in an effective and positive way. This may result in lowering, rather than inadvertently increasing, anxiety and exacerbating the situation. Their respect for their child can also increase as they can appreciate more the gains he has made when they realise what he has had to overcome in order to do so.

Information sessions, courses, conferences are all obvious ways of finding out more. Reading is another, but it can be particularly useful not only to read books about autism but books written by people who have autism or Asperger syndrome, eg Temple Grandin. These can give particular insights of how things seem from the person with autism's/Asperger syndrome's point of view. Trying to suspend one's own particular interpretations and listen to or observe your child or others with this disability can also provide surprising insights, to those who can be open enough to see them.

There are rewards

Having a child with autism or Asperger syndrome is not all difficult however. People with autism or Asperger syndrome often have an innocence and uncomplicated affection which is touching. They do not scheme, plot, rebel or undermine. We know of very few cases of a person with autism who used illicit drugs, and overdoses are also rare. If the person with autism or Asperger syndrome makes progress, this can be a source of great satisfaction and pride.

What is it like for siblings?

Many of the difficulties experienced by parents will to a greater or lesser degree be experienced by the siblings of the person with autism, and may place various restrictions on them.

For the siblings of the more able child with autism the problems can be greater than for those for example of a child with Down's syndrome. Because their brother or sister does not look disabled their socially inappropriate behaviour or naivety may attract greater ridicule.This can be a source of great embarrassment and may be felt particularly strongly during adolescence, when self-consciousness is high even for the teenager with 'normal siblings'. This will always be difficult of course but can be eased considerably if the child has already formed an accepting relationship with their sibling who has autism.

A number of factors will influence this, including the degree to which the person with autism or Asperger syndrome is affected and their particular behaviour patterns or difficulties and also the personalities of both the person and their siblings. One key factor can be the attitude of the parents.

A brother/sister of a person with autism is more likely to accept their sibling's difficulties and achieve a positive relationship with them:

- When parents can talk openly about their brother or sister's disability and encourage the children to talk openly about their feelings and accept the negative as well as the positive ones

- if they feel they have a choice about taking part in any caring that is necessary and don't always feel that they must have their sibling in tow

- and if they feel that they get their share of attention, even if it is not as much as they would like.

If the relationship is a good one, while sacrifices may need to be made there can be benefits to both. The person with autism may benefit:

- from increased manageable social opportunities with 'built-in' support

- from someone who can take their side if parents are too over protective

- from a role model nearer their age who can advise about such things as dress and hairstyle, and so on.

Their sibling can enjoy the simple acceptance they receive in return – one mother described her son as 'his sister's greatest fan', which though said as a joke very much summed up his attitude towards his sister. They may also gain satisfaction from and take pride in their brother or sister's achievements. Moreover while there can be adverse long term effects on siblings of children with a disability the bulk of research evidence suggests that this is not so in the majority of cases (Smeardon, 1998) and in fact there can be marked benefits, many showing a greater level of maturity, tolerance, and care for and awareness of others than their peers. A number also go on to enter one of the caring professions.

Groups for siblings exist in some areas. As for the parent groups, information can be obtained from The National Autistic Society.

A further concern for siblings as they get older may be whether their own children may be affected. As already shown this is a very complex area and it may be wise to seek genetic counselling if this becomes an issue.

What is the social disability in Asperger syndrome?

Studies of loneliness indicate that two rather distinct kinds of isolation contribute to it.

Social isolation

Social isolation results from people feeling that they do not occupy sufficient, or sufficiently important, roles in the social groups in which they live. This might occur through lack of availability, as is the case for people who have recently moved, or for people who live in some institutions. It might arise through avoidance of social contact, as with people who are painfully shy or as with some kinds of mental illness. Or it may be that one's life situation disrupts social contact, as, for example, is the case with the recently divorced. This kind of loneliness may afflict both people with Asperger syndrome and the parents of the child with Asperger syndrome if the latter's behaviour is socially disruptive and requires a lot of supervision.

Emotional isolation

The other kind of loneliness comes about from feeling that no-one is your friend and can be called emotional isolation. It is emotional isolation that can lead to depression and other psychiatric problems. Emotional isolation results from a perceived lack of close relationships. A wish to be close to another person is a pre-requisite for a social relationship, as is the ability to differentiate one person from another.

Whereas people with Asperger syndrome do like to be with certain people, they show less strong attachment to people, than people who are not autistic. This is apparent in the reaction of the infant to strangers, to separation from parents and in the reactions of older people with Asperger syndrome to loss. One mother, for example, reported that when she was taken to hospital in an ambulance because she had developed chest pain, her son's only question was, 'When will dinner be?' People with autism who are severely disabled may show almost no attachments to individual people but it would be wrong to conclude that this is so for people with Asperger syndrome.

Many parents feel that their child responds to their feelings for them, and shows some degree of concern about them. When asking people with Asperger syndrome specifically about this, it was found that they did mostly say that they would be upset if their mother was upset. However, for about half these individuals this was only because they would assume that their mother was upset with them.

People with Asperger syndrome do not lack emotional responsiveness. They will become distressed if a routine changes or if a specially prized object becomes lost or misplaced. It would also be wrong to assume that all people with autism or Asperger syndrome fail to differentiate between things and people. Aloofness, or indifference to social contact, is not a universal feature of autism or Asperger syndrome and most people with Asperger syndrome want, sometimes desperately, to have friends.

Van Krevelen has contrasted the dog-like attachments that people who are not autistic form with individuals, to the cat-like attachments that the person with autism or Asperger syndrome forms to situations and to people as unindividualised animals. This points up one possible source of the social disability of the person with autism or Asperger syndrome, that they lack the ability to personalise. A stroked cat does show pleasure but the same signs of pleasure that can be evoked by sunlight, or by a warm duvet. Dogs behave towards people in ways which are never shown towards objects. They have a specific set of behaviours reserved for this kind of interaction.

Theory of mind

It would undoubtedly be wrong to pursue this analogy too far, but it does illustrate what might be affected in the social functioning of the person with Asperger syndrome. People with Asperger syndrome may have a diminished understanding of that kind of thing which is unique to people (as compared to say, a robot), or they may not be able to behave or to respond to the behaviour which is unique to social situations. The first possibility has received some support from experiments reviewed by Uta Frith (1989). Simon Baron-Cohen, Alan Leslie and Frith have carried out several experiments with young children to explore what conception children had of the minds of other people.

In one case, the person conducting the experiment shows the child two dolls, Sally and Anne and with the two dolls present, Anne puts a marble into Sally's basket. Sally is then removed from the scene, and Anne moves the marble from Sally's basket to her own box. Sally is then returned and the child is asked where Sally thinks the marble is. Normal four year olds do not hesitate in saying 'the basket', ie where Sally would have seen the marble being hidden and would therefore have believed it to be. Most of the children with learning disabilities other than autism who were tested, also said that Sally would think that the marble was in the basket. The children with autism, however, expected Sally to look for it in the box where it actually was. Baron-Cohen et al, interpret this result as indicating that children with autism are less able to attribute beliefs to other people, and consider that it is evidence of a more general failure to grasp that other people have minds. This explanation of the social disability, that people with autism behave abnormally or respond abnormally to people as opposed to things, has also been the subject of an article in *Communication* by Peter Hobson (1986).

The behaviour which is especially appropriate to people, and which is never appropriately shown to objects, is communicative behaviour, or behaviour which carries a message. The communicative behaviour with which we are most familiar is speaking. Some people with autism do have difficulties with speech, but, as already noted, more able people with autism or Asperger syndrome often lose them as they get older, and people with Asperger syndrome and other autistic-like disorders may not have them at all.

Communication

Learning to speak requires a person to have the ability to memorise and recall a large number of sound and sight patterns (words) and organise the words according to arbitrary grammatical rules. Most disorders of language involve a disorder of this faculty. People with Asperger syndrome, however, do not seem to have this problem; at least, they do not lack the ability to memorise and recall words or colours, although they are less able than people who are not autistic to remember meaningful sequences. Meaning, according to the philosopher Wittgenstein, comes down to words being associated with the circumstances in which other people use the same words. The first words of most children, 'mom' or 'da-da' are associated with relationships. This suggests that the normal route for learning to speak requires that the infant has already been able to make a social relationship.

The relationship which the non-speaking infant makes must necessarily be communicated wordlessly. It seems likely that a separate communicative apparatus is used for this. The 'rules' of non-verbal communication are not taught, yet they are constantly in use in social interactions at all ages. Although there are non-verbal languages, for example American Sign Language, this earliest kind of non-verbal communication is not like a language. It has no signs for 'no' or 'yes', 'here', or 'there', 'me' or 'you'. These come later, and are learned in the same way, and usually at the same time as are the words 'no', 'yes' and so on. In adulthood, this early type of non-verbal communication is apparent mainly in the expression and interpretation of emotion: in knowing when someone is worried, for example, or in showing discomfort or pleasure to other people. Although such expressions can be deliberately produced, they are mostly 'instinctive' as are the emotional responses we make to other people. Tony Attwood (Frith, 1985; Attwood, 1985) has demonstrated that people with autism use non-emotional gestures, the kind that are learned in later life along with speech but do not use these earlier, 'instinctive' gestures. In my own study (Tantam), which was of more able people with autism, I found that some facial expressions were used normally by people with autism but that in normal conversation their faces did not register a play of feeling as the faces of people who are not autistic, do.

Other types of non-verbal expression are affected in autism. Gestures are rare and when they do occur, may appear odd because they do not appear to fit in with what the person with autism or Asperger syndrome is doing. Eye contact may also be odd, not least because some people with autism or Asperger syndrome look fixedly at another person when they are talking; people who are not autistic usually make eye contact when they are ready to stop talking.

Peter Hobson found that people with autism also had difficulties in interpreting facial expressions, and in interpreting other aspects of people and animals, such as age. He points out that an appreciation of an animal's age, like an appreciation of an animal's emotional state, is more a matter of 'an aaaah reaction .. than a cool intellectual appraisal' (Hobson 1986 p15).

If these studies are on the right lines, we are in the position to make a preliminary formulation of the social disability in autism and Asperger syndrome. It involves both an inability to appreciate that people have special characteristics and an inability to use or interpret the particular kind of non-verbal communication which is called into play in interactions between people, especially when these interactions involve feelings. Non-verbal communication appears to be based on rhythmic patterns of synchronised actions, and since the normal child uses these to pick out key words in heard speech, these rhythmic patterns also appear to act as a key to speech.

A precise understanding of the autistic disability, is, of course, very helpful in teaching, parenting or working with children with autism and Asperger syndrome. The perspective on the disability advanced here implies that people with Asperger syndrome are going to have special difficulties in situations where there is a lot of emotion, where there are important differences in social status, or where there is a discrepancy between what people are saying and what they are communicating to each other non-verbally. It is implicit in what has been said that people with autism benefit from detailed verbal explanation with things being spelt out rather than implied. Tony Attwood (1986,1998) has considered how these principles could be applied both in teaching and parenting.

What causes autism and Asperger syndrome?

Psychological

Whether or not autism and Asperger syndrome is a reaction to parental behaviour, and thus curable by an alteration in that behaviour, is a perennial question. It is a debate which, like that concerning a family cause for adult schizophrenia a decade ago, attracts partisans. To say that autism has a physical basis is assumed by one faction to imply a dismissal of any kind of psychosocial influence on cause, and to imply a hopeless prognosis. To say that psychological factors contribute to autism is assumed by the other faction to be tantamount to saying that it is the parents' fault. This latter is a particularly damaging accusation since the parents of children with autism or Asperger syndrome are so easily overwhelmed by guilt.

The style of parenting (and teaching) that a person with autism or Asperger syndrome receives can influence their behaviour for good or ill. Parents who are neither too tolerant nor too intolerant of abnormal behaviour, for example, may minimise this behaviour. The emotional security of the family may also affect the later emotional health of the person with autism or Asperger syndrome and possibly the potential to behave in an antisocial manner.

However, there are many reasons to think that children with autism or Asperger syndrome have abnormalities from infancy, and possibly from birth, that these are different from all the other problems that emotionally deprived children have, and that these abnormalities are associated with other disorders with a definite physical basis. The present balance of the evidence very strongly points to the basic disability in autism always being caused by brain disorder.

Physical

There are a variety of disorders which are associated with autism in people with learning disabilities, but it is not known whether these disorders are particularly associated with autism or the learning disability.

Physical disorders associated with Asperger syndrome are less common. However a number have been reported. They include biochemical abnormalities which may have been present during development in the womb, abnormalities of the structure of the brain which may indicate abnormal brain development, and impairment of vision or of movement which may affect a baby's interaction with its mother from birth. There are also some hereditary conditions which occur more often in the families of people with autism and may indicate a genetic basis for abnormal brain development leading to Asperger syndrome. More information about these causes can be found in Gillberg, C & Coleman, M (1996).

Biochemical abnormalities include an abnormality of the metabolism of amino-acids, one of the building blocks of proteins (amino-aciduria) and, speculatively, abnormalities of thyroid metabolism. The thyroid gland regulates metabolism and if it is not fully functioning during pregnancy, the affected child may be born with a learning disability. Milder degrees of low function in the mother or in the child have been reported, and may be more common in autism.

Structural abnormalities of the brain may be apparent in the newest part of the mid-brain, the cerebellar vermis, and affecting various parts of the brain in conditions like tuberose sclerosis and neurofibromatosis in which abnormal lumps of tissue develop and displace normal brain tissue. Epilepsy which is often taken to indicate structural abnormality of the brain is more common in autism than it is in the general population.

Visually impaired children may be more likely to develop autism, as may children with motor abnormalities. There is an association of autism with 'floppy children syndrome', and also with amyotrophic sclerosis. Both of these conditions, through either lax ligaments or muscular weakness, delay the age at which children can hold up their neck or sit without support.

A sizeable number of men with learning disabilities have an abnormality of their X chromosome which was displayed when the chromosome was incubated in a medium low in a vitamin, folic acid. These 'fragile X' chromosomes were reported to be especially common in men with autism, but this has recently been disputed. At the moment, it seems unlikely that autism, in the absence of other learning disabilities anyway, is associated with fragile X. However, attention has recently turned to another chromosome, chromosome 15, abnormalities of which may be associated with autism. There is also a familial association between bipolar affective disorder, a mental illness in which people suffer highs and lows of mood swing, and Asperger syndrome. Bipolar disorder is hereditary suggesting a possible link between its inheritance and that of autism.

Autism itself runs in families and in these families there may also be increased speech or language delay and of mild Asperger-like characteristics. It used to be thought that transmission was more often from father to son, but this probably reflects the extent to which women's superior social skills may mask mild Asperger syndrome.

Some abnormalities found in people with autism may reflect consequences of the condition and not its cause. A recent hypothesis is that people with autism have an abnormally high level of a chemical substance, serotonin, in their blood and another that they have abnormally low levels of other endogenous transmitter substances which exist in the brain to allow messages to be conducted from one nerve cell to another. However, if other psychiatric disorders are a guide, it is unlikely that these abnormalities, even if they are specifically associated with autism, will prove to be more than a bio-chemical reflection of the disordered brain function which parallels the behaviour disorder associated with autism.

There are good reasons for investigating people with Asperger syndrome even if no treatable cause for the disorder can be found. Doctors need to have as much knowledge as possible about possible causes.

What can be done for the more able person with autism or Asperger syndrome?

Improvement over time

Some people with autism or Asperger syndrome show gradual but definite improvement with age, and a very few recover almost completely. Sometimes this occurs after an apparent worsening during adolescence and early adulthood, a time of turmoil for many able people with autism or Asperger syndrome.

Why there should be an improvement is not known. It could be that the abnormality in the brain is reversible in some cases, or that other areas of the brain take over the function of the damaged area. There are probably many causes of brain abnormalities leading to autism and Asperger syndrome, and possibly several types of brain abnormality may have this effect. What happens with one of the diseases that causes autism may not apply to another. Lacking even the basic information, it is not surprising that no method of removing the basic disability by restoring brain function is known. It does appear, however, that education in two closely related areas, communication and socialisation, may accelerate improvement in some people with autism or Asperger syndrome.

Teaching social and communication skills

Education involves assessing the deficits of particular children and providing remedial training in these areas as well as opportunities to practise the newly acquired skills. Education so defined may continue after school but the bulk occurs at school.

Social and communicative skills are not consciously learnt by most people but rather are picked up during the course of social interaction. Many people with Asperger syndrome are able to pick things up in this way too but with considerable difficulty, since much social interaction seems mystifying to them. Imagine learning a new skill – skiing say. While a very young child may learn to ski by just doing it with more expert parents, an adult beginner, put into a group of expert skiers, would just be bemused. The adult's answer is to get instruction and, in the initial stage, to ski following these instructions. The person with Asperger syndrome in a group of expert social actors seems bemused too but the more able person with Asperger syndrome can, once he has developed the ability to use abstract concepts, similarly use learnt rules to guide him.

Language learning may be delayed even in the more able person with autism or Asperger syndrome and specific help may be required. Speech therapy may be useful for articulation difficulties which can themselves obstruct communication and speech therapists may also help to pinpoint areas of language difficulty. Children with autism are often delayed in learning verbal labels for objects (nouns) but are even more delayed in learning words for actions (verbs). They may also have grammatical difficulties but they are particularly delayed in learning how to form sentences to perform different actions, such as asking questions or making requests. Language learning therefore has to take place in the wider context of the social use of language. Concepts that are accessible to the child must be taught in a familiar social situation, building on any social interaction that the child has achieved. Rote learning of words is no longer considered a desirable approach to language teaching, not least because the apparent facility in language which results, can easily outrun understanding. Echolalia, stereotypy or inattention may result.

The ability to construct sentences correctly and to use and define words is only one aspect of speaking. People with autism or Asperger syndrome continue to have considerable difficulties knowing how and when to say things long after they know what to say. Teaching these 'pragmatic' aspects of language (social skills training) in the classroom may have only limited value because the person with Asperger syndrome finds it difficult to generalise from that situation to a problematic situation outside school. However, teaching conducted in the problem situation itself may be more effective although the lessons learnt may still be restricted to that situation, and not carry over to later problems. People with Asperger syndrome may benefit from being given simple rules and strategies for social interaction and may find trying these rules out in role plays useful. As with language learning, it is important not to over-estimate comprehension, however.

Emotional expressiveness

Although one basic disability in Asperger syndrome may be an abnormality of emotional expression, systematic training of emotional expressiveness has never been carried out in people with Asperger syndrome. It is not possible therefore, to say whether this would be effective. Children with autism or Asperger syndrome are often taught about facial expressions but usually using pictures rather than people.

To our knowledge there has never been an evaluation of training children with autism or Asperger syndrome to interpret others' non-verbal expressions and to be more non-verbally expressive themselves. Children who are not autistic almost never receive any instruction of this kind because they do not need it but it could be of benefit to the person with Asperger syndrome.

Social interaction

A few people with autism or Asperger syndrome, usually the least disabled, actively seek out other people's company. Although their behaviour may be gauche and occasionally a touch embarrassing, it is important that they are encouraged. Most find it only too easy to avoid interaction with other people by absorption in some other activity, often one with a stereotyped character.

Since so much learning is socially mediated, it is important that the social interactions of people with Asperger syndrome are structured in such a way that the tendency to withdraw is minimised. Withdrawal is likely to be one means of dealing with anxiety or frustration, and simply preventing withdrawal without dealing with the tension producing it may not, in the long run, be in the interests of the person with autism.

Methods to prevent withdrawal include aversion therapy (unpleasant stimulation following withdrawal), holding therapy (one or more people restraining the child physically until the child yields), or even the simple technique of demanding the child's attention. They may cause obvious distress but they can be effective in reducing the amount of social withdrawal and stereotyped behaviour for some time after, at least in that particular situation. It cannot be assumed, however, that this results in an improvement in the child's relationships. These treatments cannot be recommended while their effectiveness is unknown and they remain ethically questionable. Other, less stressful opportunities for the child with autism or Asperger syndrome to have physical contact with other people may be worth considering: sport is one such example.

The more able person with autism or Asperger syndrome is not oblivious to social situations and will respond to praise and encouragement although this may not be obvious at the time. He will also have feelings about other people although these may also be expressed indirectly, for example by an increase in stereotyped behaviour. Social contact can be increased by increasing the rewards for socialising and diminishing the reward of asocial behaviour. The speed of this process will depend on the person himself. People with Asperger syndrome who are extremely tense in social situations will need to give vent to this tension in stereotyped or asocial activity; intervention will only make matters worse. A less tense person may accept intrusion if that is accompanied by social reassurance.

Some more able people with autism or Asperger syndrome may in fact desire help to overcome such social difficulties of which they are only too aware. Given the opportunity they may work actively with a counsellor or support worker to explore their anxieties and establish strategies for coping with such situations.

Self-esteem

In contrast to the less able, the more able person with autism or Asperger syndrome is often only too aware that they have certain difficulties. This obviously impacts on their own feelings of self-worth. Too often this is compounded by the negative reactions of others. They may even feel they need to 'put on an act of being normal' in order to be accepted. This can of course be very stressful. Even when it is completely successful, which is rarely the case, it can reinforce the idea that they 'as themselves' are unacceptable.

Anxiety can be a major factor of life for the person with Asperger syndrome. This may be particularly heightened in their teens or twenties, which as already suggested, is a time of considerable change and when awareness of their differences and difficulties may be increased. They may also find at this stage that for various reasons they cannot fulfil previous expectations, perhaps of a certain career or of marrying and having a family, and so experience an increased sense of failure.

Wherever possible it is important to involve the person in their own problem-solving, dealing with anxieties and so on. Counselling by someone who understands autism and has the benefit of not being involved with the person in any other way may help. This can provide a non-threatening environment which allows the person with Asperger syndrome both the help but also the freedom and independence they need to attempt this. Not only are they then more likely to invest in making the solutions work but this also empowers them and adds to their self-belief.

Parents and other support workers can also help by encouraging realistically achievable but high enough expectations for the person to experience success, and also seeking the right balance between giving enough support and standing back and letting the person take reasonable risks and appropriate responsibility for his own actions and decisions. If people in these roles show their respect for the person and his abilities, it is easier for him to accept appropriate help and still retain a positive sense of his own worth.

As referred to in relation to the needs of parents, early diagnosis is also a key factor for the person themselves. Doctors may delay diagnosis for fear of labelling a child. However, as one person with Asperger syndrome observed "I have been labelled a lot of things and Asperger syndrome is better than stupid, lazy, or ignorant."

Modifying behaviour

Occasionally people with Asperger syndrome behave repeatedly in some unacceptable way, and it is necessary to consider how to bring pressure to bear on them to effect a change. Common problems are repetitive questioning, imposition of a routine on other people, and aggression.

The first step in trying to modify the behaviour of the person with Asperger syndrome will almost always involve some negotiation. He should be told what the unwanted behaviour is and why it is causing a problem to other people. It is important to have some idea why the person with Asperger syndrome is behaving as he is but it is rarely possible for him to say why himself, although for the more able person a chance to explore this in counselling as outlined earlier may lead to such self awareness.

Anxiety

Anxiety is a common cause of an increase in rituals and in repetitive questioning. One boy was told by an exasperated sister that he would be 'the death of his mother'. He subsequently monopolised several medical consultations with repeated questions about how people died. Another boy pestered his mother with questions about a nuclear holocaust, even waking her at night to ask if it was going to happen. He could not be reassured but kept asking the same question over and over again. The questioning stopped when a doctor arranged to see mother and son together. The mother told her son about her own fears that her cancer of the breast (she had had a breast removed for cancer) had come back. He was then able to express his own worries about this. She had previously thought him completely unconcerned.

If relieving anxiety does not help the problem, then some kind of social control has to be considered. This is particularly likely to be needed in those cases where a person with Asperger syndrome has found that behaving in a particular, upsetting way is satisfying. People with Asperger syndrome are no more unselfish than others and there is a particular risk of this happening if parents centre their lives on their child. The first step in social control is to consider what kinds of control are acceptable to parents. Professionals sometimes encourage parents to ban their grown-up child from the home unless they mend their ways but this kind of control is rarely acceptable to the parent of a person who is handicapped. The control measure should not be an arbitrary punishment but one that is an understandable consequence of the behaviour. Very often this can be the withdrawal of some rewarding activity the parents perform for the person with Asperger syndrome – one he has come to take for granted. The measure to be adopted should then be discussed with the person with Asperger syndrome in as unemotional way as possible, along with a careful delineation of the unacceptable behaviour, so that there is no doubt in anyone's mind when these consequences will follow. It is often the case that the person with Asperger syndrome will try and dissociate himself from the procedure; it may sometimes be necessary to put things in writing.

If it is not one but many behaviours which are the problem, then the sort of approach outlined above may not work. And, if the unacceptable behaviour is a new phenomenon this may indicate there are stresses in the living or working situation such that the help of a social worker or doctor may be indicated. Socially unacceptable behaviour may be symptomatic of a mood disorder or other mental illness, and a medical assessment may be particularly helpful if there is any suspicion of this.

Mental illness and Asperger syndrome

Mental illness is much more common than people often assume, and people with Asperger syndrome are certainly not immune. Clinicians are often of the opinion that more able people with autism or Asperger syndrome are particularly vulnerable, especially during adolescence and early adulthood. Epilepsy may also begin at this time but this seems to be less common in more able than in more disabled people with autism.

The most common mental illnesses affecting people with Asperger syndrome are depression or anxiety states. They may cause alterations in behaviour but are accompanied by the same symptoms of loss of appetite, difficulty with sleep, and lack of concentration with which they are associated in other people. Treatments which are effective for anxiety or depression in people who are not autistic are also effective in people with autism or Asperger syndrome. As long as they realise this, general practitioners and psychiatrists with no special experience of autism or Asperger syndrome can be of considerable assistance in remedying these mood disorders.

Some people with Asperger syndrome suffer from regular fluctuations of mood which sometimes become extreme and need hospital treatment. Occasionally they may hear voices or develop a false conviction when in this state. The usual treatments for this condition of manic-depressive psychosis also apply in autism or Asperger syndrome, and, again, psychiatrists who know this can do a lot to help with this emergency even if they have no special experience of autism or Asperger syndrome.

Long-term treatment with lithium or other drugs is sometimes effective in preventing illness recurring.

Schizophrenia is another serious mental illness in which people hear voices, have difficulty in thinking clearly, or develop fantastic convictions. Autism is not the same as schizophrenia but a few people with autism or Asperger syndrome do seem to develop this condition as well. They may then need long-term tranquillisers to prevent a relapse. It should, however, be emphasised that long-term tranquillisers are not an effective treatment for the autism or Asperger syndrome alone.

People with Asperger syndrome often become less disabled as they get older

Many people with autism are too disabled to make substantial progress but for those who do not have serious language difficulties or learning disabilities (the more able group in other words), a slow reduction in their disability does seem to occur in response to normal social interaction. This reduction appears to carry on beyond the end of adolescence into adult life.

An important ingredient of this improvement is that the person with Asperger syndrome is exposed to as normal a social environment as possible. If the person with Asperger syndrome develops a serious psychiatric disorder, a serious problem with their physical health, or if their freedom is restricted because of an offence, then normal social interactions will be to some extent curtailed and social development will be slowed. If the person with Asperger syndrome is employed or in full-time education, theory says that, since the person will be brought into more contact with other people, social development will be spurred on, but no follow-up study stretches far enough into adulthood to be sure.

A few people eventually recover almost completely, but most never become completely independent. A surprising amount can, however, be achieved by the patient accumulation of social gains over a period of years.

A note on diagnosis for the professional

Kanner in 1943 and Asperger writing independently in 1944 were both struck by the amount of social detachment and self-absorption shown by some disturbed children; both applied Bleuler's terms 'autistic' to them. Both psychiatrists intended to distinguish autism from mental handicap or gross neurological disorder by restricting it to children of normal intelligence and without neurological signs. However, the term autism rapidly extended far beyond this so that numerous attempts had to be made to contain it within reasonable boundaries.

Studies of large groups of children carried out by Lorna Wing, Gillberg and others have shown that there are many children, very similar to the children described by Kanner, yet quite unlike normal children who do not quite meet all the requirements for a diagnosis of 'Kanner' syndrome.

ICD-10 and DSM-IV recognise this situation by coining the term 'pervasive developmental disorder' (PDD) and giving its characteristics as the triad of social impairment which Wing and Gould described in their epidemiological study. Other synonyms for PDD which are in common usage are 'autistic spectrum disorder' or, more simply, 'autism'. We prefer the latter terms since its original meaning of one of the core signs of schizophrenia has now become obsolete. At the moment, it seems likely that the same disability underlies all these conditions; consequently some people with a PDD may benefit from the educational and rehabilitative provisions currently found to be of benefit to some children with childhood autism.

Childhood autism is one of the pervasive developmental disorders, in which the triad of social impairment is apparent from early infancy, is more likely to be severe, and is associated with language and learning disabilities. Asperger syndrome now receives its own diagnostic recognition, but it is arguable how much value there is in differentiating a specific group of patients with Asperger syndrome since these patients differ only from those with childhood autism in having less severe disabilities, a later age of onset and less impairment of language. However, Asperger syndrome is a useful functional label for the sub-group of people with autism who are sociable, very clumsy, verbally skilled and with highly developed special interests. These people may or may not have a typical history of early childhood autism.

It would be useful to differentiate Asperger syndrome if it had a specific cause. The many studies conducted to try to differentiate Asperger syndrome from other types of autism have failed to demonstrate this, with the possible exception of the greater likelihood that Asperger syndrome is associated with clumsiness and with a family history of bipolar affective disorder.

However, it is possible to differentiate a sub-group of people with Asperger syndrome who are demonstrably odd in their manner and appearance, from those who do not appear markedly odd but do seem immature. The former group probably include people whose main communicative difficulty is with social and emotional expression. The latter may include a majority of people whose main difficulties in non-verbal communication lie in their problems in interpreting or understanding emotional and social cues. This group may have some of the greatest deficits of empathy of all sufferers from PDD, and may be the most likely to come into conflict with others as a result.

The diagnosis of autism or Asperger syndrome can only be made with confidence after a thorough development history concentrating on social, motor and communicative development, reactions to other people, reactions to objects, response to change, and play and interest patterns has been taken. Many developmental abnormalities characteristic of autism or Asperger syndrome are also shown by normal children and, when a more able autistic population is considered, some of the most typical are only shown by a few children. When making a diagnosis, it is therefore important to consider the pattern of a child's development rather than the presence or absence of a few specific behaviours.

Information about early development is not always obtainable, but a diagnosis of probable autism (including Asperger syndrome) can reasonably be made using the criteria shown in Table 3.

Table 3 Criteria for a diagnosis of probable autism in adolescence or adulthood
A All three of the following:
1 Social disability especially apparent in work and friendship
2 Markedly unusual interests, often involving collecting objects of special interest or facts in some circumscribed area.
3 Abnormal conduct of social interactions sufficient to cause difficulty in communication. Always associated with abnormal non-verbal expression, although this may be mild, this may also be expressed in a disorder of speech and in an apparent immaturity of behaviour in social situations.
B The above characteristics date from early childhood or, if this cannot be established, do not date from an episode of psychosis.

There is an advantage in making a diagnosis of autism or Asperger syndrome even in adulthood as it can help parents and others to have an insight into the specific problems facing the person with autism or Asperger syndrome. Further, it can divert blame or criticism where this is inappropriately directed at disability. It is also important to avoid a misdiagnosis of schizophrenia, which may lead to the inappropriate prescription of medication.

References

Attwood, T (1998) *Asperger's syndrome – a guide for parents and professionals.* London, Jessica Kingsley.

Ehlers, S and Gillberg, C (1993) The epidemiology of Asperger syndrome : a total population study. *Journal of Child Psychology and Psychiatry* 34: 1327–1350.

Gillberg, C and Coleman, M (1996) Autism and medical disorders: a review of the literature. *Developmental Medicine and Child Neurology* 38: 191–202.

Grandin, T and Scariano, M M (1986) *Emergence: labelled autistic*. New York, Warner Books.

Quine, L and Pahl, J (1985) Examining the causes of stress in families with severely mentally handicapped children. *British Journal of Social Work* 15(5): 501–517.

Smeardon, L (1998) All in the family – autistic spectrum disorders and sibling relationships. *Communication* Summer.

Further reading

Aston, M. (2001) *The other half of Asperger syndrome.* London, The National Autistic Society.

Atwood, T. (1993) *Why does Chris do that?* London, The National Autistic Society.

Cumine, V, Leach, J and Stevenson, G (1998) *Asperger syndrome, a practical guide for teachers*. London, David Fulton Publishers.

Datlow Smith, M, Belcher, R and Juhrs, P (1995) *A guide to successful employment for individuals with autism.* Baltimore, Paul H Brookes.

Howlin, P (1997) *Autism: preparing for adulthood.* London, Routledge.

Ives, M. (1999) *What is Asperger syndrome and how will it affect me?* London, The National Autistic Society.

Leicester City Council and Leicestershire County Council (1998) *Asperger syndrome – practical strategies for the classroom – a teacher's guide*. London, The National Autistic Society.

Mawhood, L and Howlin, P (1997) *A supported employment scheme for able adults with autism or Asperger syndrome*. London, The National Autistic Society.

Mawhood, L and Howlin, P (1997) *A supported employment scheme for able adults with autism or Asperger syndrome*. London, The National Autistic Society.

The National Autistic Society (1999) *Independent living for adults with autism and Asperger syndrome.* London, The National Autistic Society.

The National Autistic Society (1999) *What next? Moving on from diagnosis.* London, The National Autistic Society.

Wing, L (1996) *The autistic spectrum: a guide for parents and professionals*. London, Constable Publishers.